TABLE OF CONTENTS

CHAPTER 1

INTRODUCTION

First off, thanks for making the purchase! If you are in any way interested in marathon, long-distance, or endurance running, you are in the right place.

If you are a beginner and are looking for a starting point, this will benefit you greatly. But it's not just for beginners; the intermediate and advanced runner will also find some great information and inspiration in this book, I'm sure.

For many people, running a marathon is the pinnacle of their fitness career. It is the benchmark in long-distance running prowess. This is why I have focused on marathon running rather than your "everyday" track and field running.

"If you shoot for the moon and miss, you'll still end up amongst the stars"

I would like you to keep this great phrase in your mind as you read through this book. If you feel that all of the references to marathon running do not apply to you, you should revisit this quote.

Although a lot of people set out to achieve this goal, many never actually achieve it. This can be down to a number of things, but, most commonly, it is lack of correct advice. Lack of consistency, feelings of self-doubt, and incorrect mind-set also play a part in the failed attempts of many.

This book will outline the factors that will lead to your success as a long-distance/marathon runner. I believe that my personal experience, lessons I have learned and mistakes that I have made with this type of training, will help budding long-distance runners reach their goals in the most direct way possible.

Here's to your success!

CHAPTER 2

WHY SHOULD YOU TAKE MY ADVICE?

Hi, I'm Jim from JimsHealthAndMuscle.com. I am a qualified fitness coach and personal trainer. I have been into fitness for much of my life and have been at both ends of the fitness scale, from long-distance running and endurance to competition bodybuilding. I served a number of years in the British Army where I was part of an elite airborne unit—9 Parachute Squadron Royal Engineers.

As you can see, I have changed the conditioning of my body more than most.

But this book is all about endurance and long-distance running—marathons and beyond!

I know there are plenty of books out there about this type of training, but I would like to share my firsthand experience of developing from a guy who couldn't run 1.5 miles in 15 minutes to a guy who could be handed a pair of running shoes and be standing confidently at the start line of a marathon in the time it took to tie those shoes up. That was all the preparation time that I needed.

Oh, and I got to a point when I could cover the same 1.5 mile distance in 8 minutes and 22 seconds!

Let's start at the beginning.

It was summer 1999, and I had just finished my secondary school education. Not being an academic and not knowing what I wanted to do with my life, I decided to enrol for a Business Studies class at college. It wasn't long before I realised that sitting in an office was not something that I really wanted to do. (Looking back, this was a fairly good opportunity, but you live, you learn, I suppose.)

Anyway, about six months into this college education, I decided that I wanted a bit of excitement from my life and the thought of being an average Joe with a regular nine-to-five job made me pretty depressed. It was at this point that I ventured into the local army careers office.

"So, do you have any idea what you want to do as a job in the army?" asked the sergeant at the front desk.

I had heard a lot about airborne forces and the parachute regiment and wanted a piece of that.

"Yeah. I want to look at joining the paras," I said, not realising at that time that you don't simply "join the paras!"

"Okay, let's have a chat," he replied (probably thinking, "Jeez! Here's another one with absolutely no clue!")

The sergeant had a good chat with me and concluded that I should look at getting a trade in the Royal Engineers; I could then volunteer for para training at a later date. This way I would have a trade, be on higher pay, and also get to jump out of planes and serve with airborne forces.

To go down this path, however, I would need to pass the army aptitude test at a higher level than I had done.

I took this aptitude test four times with a six-week gap between tests before the sergeant just gave me a pass. (I actually think I failed the fourth time as well, but he just fixed my score. It was good to see someone give me a chance.)

So that was me going to the next stage of the army selection process. And this was the fitness testing stage!

These fitness tests were over a long weekend where all potential recruits are taken to an army training centre and tested on attitude, strength, and endurance and checked if we were medically fit.

As I was into weight training at the time, I did well with the strength tests, but, on the last day, there is a mile-and-a-half run that must be completed in something like fifteen minutes. This is very achievable and you could probably do this at a fast-paced walk.

This 1.5 mile circuit is led by a PTI (physical training instructor) who is the pace maker. If you stick with this guy, you will pass—simple!

There were about twenty guys on this stage of the selection process with me, and we all started at a steady jog close to the PTI. At about a minute into the test, my breathing was all over the place, my lower back was giving me pain, and I started to get a stitch. I must have looked like I was at the final few miles of a marathon! I remember the PTI turning to me and shouting,

"What's up, Atkinson? You got a sucking chest wound?" before laughing and leaving me to drop back behind the whole squad.

When I eventually crossed the finish line, I gave my name to one of the corporals and he noted my time down. Needless to say, this was a big fat fail, and if I did want to join the army, I would have to start some kind of running programme and sort my cardio fitness levels out before I could try this selection process again.

Back at the careers office, the same sergeant that I had originally spoken to gave me a fitness plan to follow so I could try again in six months' time.

So getting into the army wasn't as easy as I had first thought, and I was glad that I had been put on the "trade path" rather than the "parachute regiment path" at this point.

College was still in the picture, and I would get up an hour earlier each morning and run around a two-mile circuit that I had planned out. At first, this took 25 minutes, and within a few weeks, it was down to seventeen minutes—sorted!

Several months passed and the time came for my next attempt at the army selection process, and I flew through it this time, sticking with the PTI and being amongst the first to cross the finish line on the final mile and a half test.

I finally joined the army in 2001, so this had taken me the best part of two years!

CHAPTER 3

ANOTHER LEVEL OF

LONG-DISTANCE RUNNING

When my basic training was done, I was a whole lot fitter; I could run ten miles at a "steady state" pace and be reasonably comfortable.

But the time soon came when I would actually sign up to try "P-company." This is the selection process that you have to pass to be able to serve with an airborne unit. If I were to follow my original plan from my first visit to the army careers office, this is something that I would need to do.

Fitness and endurance levels are tested through basic training and second phase training in the Royal Engineers, and many recruits decide after the first two phases of their army career that to serve with 9 para squadron is way beyond their reach.

"If I struggle with these, there is no way that I would pass P-company," was the mentality.

These doubts were also at the front of my mind. It didn't help that I was told by my training staff that I would never pass!

But I decided to go ahead anyway.

I had now been in the army around twenty-four weeks only and was on my way to start "Pre para." Pre para is a five- to seven-week period that anyone from the Royal Engineers wishing to give P-company a shot must complete. This is also known as "The beat up course." In the end, there were only three of us that actually signed up. So off we went to start the training.

At the early stages of the first run that we were taken on, it became very clear that this was going to be tough!

Sure, I had progressed with my running very well, but this type of training was above and beyond what I even imagined possible.

For the next few weeks on the lead up to P-company, lots of potentials joined us and lots more dropped out. Every day we were pushed passed our limits on these long runs. It really is a good system because by the time the beat up course is finished, the engineers that are sent to actually do P-company are less likely to embarrass the corps, and there is a higher pass rate.

Anyway, I learned some very valuable lessons about endurance, stamina, and long-distance running that I know I would not have learned if I'd decided not to take up the challenge of P-company.

It is this experience that I would like to call upon and share with you in the pages of this book. I truly believe that the information that I outline here is the best way to approach marathon and progressive running training.

CHAPTER 4

HEALTH CHECK

Before you embark on any change of diet or fitness programme, please consult your doctor if you are unsure of the health implications of these changes.

If you are taking medication, please check with your doctor to make sure it is ok for you to make these changes.

If you are in any doubt at all, please check with your doctor first. It may be helpful to ask for a blood pressure, cholesterol, and weight check. You can then have these read again in a few months after exercise or change of diet to see the benefit.

CHAPTER 5

ACCOUNTABILITY: COMMIT TO YOUR GOAL

Nothing gets you more motivated than having a deadline and a timescale! This is why I would advise that as soon as you decide that you want to run a marathon or a half marathon, or you decide you just want to get better at running, you should sign up for a race or set yourself a personal deadline.

If you do want to sign up for a race, but this is a year or two away and you can't sign up yet, you should find out the earliest possible date that you can and mark it on your calendar.

It's all well and good saying that you will do something like this, but you won't be half as committed to your goal if you don't have this type of accountability. It really is a great tool.

We are all guilty of not committing to certain things at times, and if there is no deadline, where's the urgency? We could just call off our plans for today and aim to complete them tomorrow.

But as Apollo Creed screams to Rocky in the film Rocky III when he is slacking:

"There is no tomorrow!"

The problem is that not everyone has an Apollo Creed looking over their shoulder for motivation and accountability!

You will know if you are actually serious about achieving this goal when it comes to actually signing up for a marathon. Of course, you are probably thinking that you will sign up when you feel a bit more "ready," but guess what? You will never feel ready, so if you do want to run a full marathon or even a half marathon, get your application filled in.

If you fail the first time, chalk it up as "good experience" and get back on the horse! You will be better prepared for your next attempt.

CHAPTER 6

CHOOSE YOUR SHOES... OR GO BAREFOOT?

Which footwear you will run in is a very important decision that you will need to make. There are many respectable sports brands out there that will appeal to you right away.

Although these brands do offer some good running footwear, they also offer training equipment that is oriented towards fashion rather than function. And you should be looking for function over anything else.

You could just go over to Amazon or eBay and pick up some running shoes at discounted prices. But this is a risk. Sure, you may end up with a set of running shoes that are perfect for you, but you could also end up with some that will cause you problems.

Personally, I advise any runner to go for a "road running"/general purpose shoe. You can buy "Off road"/trail shoes and also "track" shoes. The advantages of good road running shoes are that they will have good cushioning and a shallow hard-wearing tread, and they will be light.

These attributes will help to protect from the impact that your body will be exposed to during your running training. Since I found my first decent pair of running shoes, I have stuck to the same brand and model. Now I would not suggest for a second that this brand and model are the best for everyone, because everyone is different. For example, there are runners who will "over pronate" their feet, and there are other runners who will "under pronate" their feet when running. This means that some runners will need a shoe that fits slightly differently or they will need a special insole.

It is for this reason that I cannot suggest a certain make or model of shoe for you. If you are serious about getting the best running shoes for your current running style, it is a good idea to go to a

professional running store and ask for their advice.

I do know that the best stores will have you jog on a treadmill so they can look at your natural foot strike and offer you the best running shoes that suit your style.

By all means, look into this as much as you can. The time spent researching will not be wasted.

Some of the best brands that I have had experience with are Asics, Mizuno, and Saucony, so these may be good places to start.

Researching and buying a good set of running shoes is great for an entry into the running world and the financial investment that comes with it is well worth it. But I would like to mention at this point that these days, there is a big movement towards "Barefoot" running. There is a lot to be said about this subject and I believe that there are many in-depth books and a lot of information out there now that cover the pros and cons of this idea.

When I first heard of barefoot running, as I suppose many people do, I thought of running with no shoes on at all. As you can imagine, running over gravel or on roads may become fairly uncomfortable to say the least. But the whole idea of running barefoot is not to test your resolve when it comes to running across harsh terrain, but rather to change your running style so that you are able to run for longer, decrease chance of injury and become more efficient.

Although it is called "Barefoot running", you can actually buy "Barefoot running" shoes. This may sound like a contradiction in terms but it is the physiological theory and practice that makes barefoot running what it is rather than the literal sense of the phrase.

The main idea behind barefoot running is that you have a "zero drop heel". Traditionally, most footwear including running shoes have a raised heel. Needless to say, a raised heel actually causes a heel strike when walking and running.

Most people have learned to walk and run with these raised heeled shoes and as a result, they have developed a posture and function that relies on this support.

How does a raised heel cause problems? Well, the theory suggests that the raised heel throws off the natural alignment of the body which has an effect on the spine and ultimately general posture will be effected. It is fact that bad posture can cause many problems throughout the body.

When running in a raised heel shoe, you will also rely on a heel strike as a natural and comfortable means of running. Running in this manner causes more shock to the knees and hip joints as the leg is effectively bought to a stop every time the heel hits the ground.

It is for this reason that many running shoe manufacturers have developed shoes that are designed to take this shock away with extra cushioning and shock absorbing technology. This often makes the heel of the shoe a little bit bigger still.

The barefoot running method teaches a different style of running altogether that addresses the shock problem by changing the way the runner actually runs, rather than using additional support and technology to counter this potentially damaging stress.

In short, the barefoot runner will develop a style of running that reduces heel strike to a "heel graze". This puts more focus on the calf muscles and almost completely takes away the shock from heel strike that is focused on the knee.

As a staunch advocate of the correct use of kinesiology and physiology, when it comes to fitness and exercise of any kind, I am totally on board with the general theory of barefoot running and I would advise most people to at least give it some consideration and not just dismiss the idea.

Although I don't feel qualified to offer detailed information on barefoot running, I would like to offer one word of warning, and this is a big one; If you do decide to go ahead and try this, you should know that it is not a style of running that you can simply switch to, especially if you have already developed a running style in traditional running shoes. It is very sensible to treat this as a project and you should adopt the approach of learning to walk again.

Compared to many barefoot runners, I have only dabbled in this practice myself but I can confirm from my limited experience that this style of running does indeed take the shock away from the knees, it is addictive, it feels right (for me at least) and the long term benefits are very plausible. But you should spend time learning and practicing the "barefoot running form" and transition slowly introducing short barefoot running sessions into your running training routine.

I can also confirm that any warnings that you might hear about a slow transition from traditional running footwear to barefoot running footwear are to be taken extremely seriously.

On receiving my first set of barefoot running shoes (Vibram five fingers), I couldn't wait to get out there and put these to the test. I

had originally planned to do a short two mile run so that I could practice my new running form in conjunction with testing out my new functional (but strange looking) barefoot running shoes.

As soon as I had started running, I loved the new feel. Everything about this running style was great, it was liberating, I felt more connected to the ground, I felt more agile and the whole running experience felt like it flowed better. Six miles into my planned two mile run, I had finished!

At first, I just thought that my calves felt like they had taken a battering, but nothing that I wasn't used to. After all, I had just finished a six mile run and these muscles were not used to being worked in this way, so it was expected.

One week later and I was still struggling with pain in my Achilles tendon. It turned out that I had overdone it and that I should have listened to the warnings and I should not have gone against my own judgement.

As mentioned before; I do not have extensive experience in this area and I haven't achieved anything special in this area but I do believe that it is worth looking into. Barefoot running is probably not for everyone, but I feel that the theories that back up the practice are very solid and it should not be dismissed.

Moving forward, I plan to continue working with this running form and learn the ins and outs of it for myself and hopefully be able to report on the long term effects at a later date.

Until then, I would suggest that you have a look at this theory too, give it a try and consider the benefits, but please heed the warnings.

So after all that, what is the best cause of action? Do you buy some traditional running shoes or do you start barefoot running? Well, this is what I suggest; You should do both. If you have always worn traditional foot ware that has any type of heel on it, then you should make it a priority to acquire some traditional running shoes. Make sure that these are good quality and if possible, you should have your personal running pattern tested by an authority if you wish to get optimal results on your first shot.

I would also advise that you look into the barefoot theory and give it a try, but I can't stress enough that you should take the transition slowly. An injury can set you back more than just a week or two. If you are a total beginner who has always worn a traditional shoe and heal however, I would advise that you focus on getting started with a running routine and put the barefoot ideas and aspirations on the shelf for now. As a beginner, the last thing that you need is too much information and contradiction.

CHAPTER 7

WHERE TO START

This section is really aimed at the beginner, but it may still hold some useful information for the veteran.

With anything that you do, you have to start from the beginning, and I firmly believe that having a solid foundation to build on is a must if you want results.

It would be great if every goal that you had was achievable overnight, but with any serious fitness goal, the mind-set of progressional training is a fundamental factor for success!

Of course, you would not expect to be able to run a marathon in a few short weeks of training. And I would like to make it clear that if you are just starting out, there is a long road ahead of you… (Excuse the pun.)

This may sound negative, and many people would be put off by the fact that at least six months of hard, consistent, and smart training will only get them a small step closer to their goal.

I'm talking about the guys that have never done any exercise before and would like to take up the challenge of a marathon.

If you are this guy or gal, I would first like to congratulate you on making this decision and also like to reassure you that you CAN do this.

When you cross that finish line, I'm sure that it will be one of the greatest accomplishments of your life, and your training, character building, and determination leading up to this accomplishment will definitely enrich you as a person.

YOUR FIRST RUN (WHAT TO EXPECT)

The first time you step out of your door, you will probably be motivated, have some shiny new running shoes and training attire, and be ready to start pounding the pavement.

There are a few things that can literally kill your motivation and make you hang up your new running shoes permanently if you are not careful. The biggest killer of your goals in this situation is...

"too much, too soon."

I have seen it, overheard conversations about it, and actually been there myself.

Everything's great. You are all ready to start your marathon training, you have planned your route, you are hydrated, and you know this is going to be the start of something very special! You give a few cursory hamstring stretches and set off on your first run.

Two minutes in and you are fighting for air, your lungs are on fire, you feel sick, and you are wondering how on god's green earth you are even going to finish your first run when you are in this state and you can still see your front door?

Believe me; if you have never felt this way before, you need to actually be there to understand the mental effect that this has on you. It can be devastating!

You will no doubt be able to relate to this feeling very soon as your training progresses. But I will say that it can be controlled, and when you look back at these events, they won't seem that bad. It's just while you are there that you will feel your world is ending!

Before you start your training, please read the Breathing and Running Style chapters. If you can understand and practice this before you even start your first run, it will help you out massively.

YOUR FIRST RUN (WHAT TO DO)

Once you have your breathing and running style sorted, you will be ready for your first run.

The thing is, your first run will not actually be a run! Remember that this is all about progression and you have to start somewhere. If you have never been on a run before, your body isn't used to the kind of stresses put on it, so you will probably end up in the state that we just talked about.

Once you have your route planned out, you should don your trainers and get ready, as you would expect. But your first training session should be a steady walk around your route. This will benefit you more than you probably think.

First of all, it will start you on your routine. Next, it will get you used to your new running shoes. These are a vital piece of kit for any runner.

"Bad shoes = Bad feet, and with bad feet, you can't do a whole lot of running"

Another thing that walking your route will help you with is getting your body used to prolonged activity. These early sessions will also help you to prepare mentally for your training too as you will be able to visualise your route and you will get to know how long this will take you or how close you are to the finish line.

Depending on how fit you are or how quickly you progress, you may want to do this walk for the first full week, but you can assess your progress after your first session.

All that being said, starting off slowly is one thing, but progression is vital if you want to improve and actually reach "long-distance runner status."

This "easy start" approach may be refreshing to some readers, but you also need to progress and push yourself. It may take you a few weeks to find your limits and assess your fitness progression, but this is all part of the process. It is important that you find the right balance.

This is what I would do if I had never done any fitness:

First Session
• Walk my route at a consistent pace

Second Session
• If the previous session was too easy, I would pick up my pace a bit.
• If the previous session was too hard, I would shorten the route a bit.
• If the previous session made me out of breath slightly and had me sweating but I was otherwise comfortable, I would consider a short jogging stint at the last section of my next session.

As you can see, there are a few factors that you can change each time that you train. The important part at this stage is to never sit back and go through the motions; you MUST be progressing. If your sessions do not push you slightly, you will not develop the endurance that you are looking for.

But at this point, there is no need to get to the stage of physical discomfort mentioned at the beginning of this chapter. It will only mess with your mind.

EMPTY YOURSELF

It is common knowledge that you must not eat a big meal before you train in this game, but it is not common knowledge that running with a "full tank" can cause you problems. I understand that this may make me sound crude, but I think it is well worth mentioning. You can thank me for it later!

Before you start any run, you should go to the toilet. This kind of physical activity can bring on a call of nature very suddenly!

Like I said, you can thank me for this little gem later.

SUMMARY
Here is a list of things that you should take the time to do before you set out on your first training session;

• Plan your route: Make sure you have a route that is at least 1 mile long (You can choose any distance, but it should take you at least thirty minutes to complete at this point). A good idea when planning this route is to have it as a circuit starting and ending in the same place.

• Get a good pair of running shoes (see "Choose your Shoes" section of this book).

• Familiarize yourself with the following chapters: "Breathing" and "Running style."

• Don't forget to go to the toilet!

CHAPTER 8

RUNNING STYLE

When you are new to running, it may seem simple. All you have to do is put on some running shoes and start running. You will get better the more that you do it, right? This is partly true, but any veteran will tell you that there is a lot more to it than you would think. We will get around to covering some of the more important factors in the various chapters of this book.

Incorrect running style can have a negative effect on your progress and, more importantly, on your health. So it is important that you are aware of the flaws in your natural running style so that they can be corrected.

When I first started running, I noticed that I would occasionally get pain in my lower back. At first I didn't really look into this much, as I thought it was due to an old injury from weight lifting.

About a year before I started running, I had pinched a disc in my lower back while training with weights. This was a fairly nasty injury and was down to my lack of knowledge and "hungry ego" when it came to weight lifting at the time. Another valuable lesson learned as I had problems walking without any pain for about six months.

So naturally, I put the lower back pain down to a weakness from my injury and hoped that my new running routine would strengthen and heal it over time. But one day I was running past a shop window for some reason (I normally run over fields and in a "green" setting if I can) and had to do a double take at the reflection.

My posture was horrible! I was leaning forward way too much, and I didn't at all look like a natural runner. In fact, my head and shoulders were almost in a position that made me look like I was about to fall over!

That's why people would stare at me! It wasn't my outrageously short running shorts after all! From then on, I made a conscious

effort to correct my posture on every run that I did.

This was hard and it took a lot of effort to constantly remind myself to straighten up, but eventually the new correct running position that I had trained myself to use became natural for me. Because of this change, my lower back pain totally disappeared within a few short weeks, and I was able to concentrate on my progress.

What's the correct running position then?

Although I had a problem with my upper body position when running, there are a bunch of other factors that can cause you problems.

You should study each point on this list and make sure that you are aware of the correct positioning. You may naturally have incorrect positioning in one or more areas.

If so, the earlier that you correct this, the easier it will be. My advice would be to make these corrections a priority. You should focus on this before you set out to cover personal best distances or timed running sessions.

Of course, if you are able to stay focused on your correct positioning and progress at the same time, great! But be honest with yourself, and don't slip back into bad habits just for the sake of progress.

Correct posture is more important for long-term success.

Let's start from the feet and work up:

YOUR FEET

Your toes should be pointing directly forward. Some people have a tendency to point their feet outwards or inwards.

Each time that your leading foot lands when you are running, it should hit the ground at the middle (not the heel of your foot) and also should be directly below your hips. Using a "zero drop heel" will make this a lot clearer to gauge but as mentioned in a previous chapter, a transition to this type of running shoe is advised if you are used to a traditional heeled or cushioned shoe.

YOUR ABDOMEN

You should engage your stomach muscles, pulling your belly button inwards. Make sure that you are not leaning forward or backwards.

YOUR ARMS

You can have your upper arms close to your sides with your lower arm at a right angle to the floor. As you run, you should find a comfortable swinging rhythm. I find that holding my phone, GPS or music player in one of my hands helps me to make this feel more natural.

YOUR SHOULDERS

Your shoulders should be directly above your pelvis. You can push your chest out slightly to help with this. It is also common to feel tension in your shoulders and neck, so be aware of this and shake it off if you start to feel the build-up.

YOUR HEAD

Your head should be in a position so you can view the path in front of you at eye level. It will help if you have a horizon to look at. This will help keep your airway open as well.

I will admit that most people have their own unique running style, and that's fine. I'm sure that you will develop your own individual style over time. But the points mentioned here should be used as a guide if you are unsure.

If you do start to feel aches and pains in certain areas, look again at your posture and reassess; it could be down to something mentioned here.

CHAPTER 9

BREATHING

Although I managed to condition my body to be able to run several miles in a set time and managed to get through basic training and second phase training in the army, I did not learn how to control my breathing until early on in my para training.

I feel that I should mention that when I was a kid, I did suffer with asthma. I'm not sure if I still have this now, but I do believe that my active lifestyle has probably knocked it out of me….. If that is possible?

So as you can imagine, the cardio tests and training that I got through in the army up until I reached my para selection course were achieved with sheer luck and a bit of determination. But this was not enough to pass the para selection course.

If I were sent back in time to the beginning of my long-distance running career, I would put the breathing techniques that I know of now to use right away.

STORY TIME AGAIN

At the start of the pre para selection process—"the beat up course"—the guys are pushed to their limits every day. It seemed to me that the pre para staff really wanted you to fail, and the running sessions that we would go on were brutal and like nothing I had ever done before.

Right away, my lack of understanding on how to control my breathing gave me some big problems, and with a background of asthma, I would have to sort this out quickly or be kicked off the course and not earn a maroon beret or get my para wings. I would have to spend the rest of my army career wearing a regular blue beret and be known to the airborne solders that did earn their place among

the airborne forces as a "Crap hat".

We were about a week and a half into the "beat up course" when one of the staff actually gave me the advice that I needed.

We were mid run, and he dropped back so he was running alongside of me. He didn't say anything for around ten seconds; I could just feel him staring at me as we ran.

I kept looking forward, carried on struggling to breathe and waited for the inevitable dig from him about me "not being made of the right stuff for 9 squadron" or something along those lines. I just concentrated on getting through this one run. After a while, he said, "Atkinson! Keep your head up! You're missing out on some good views around this training area. They filmed James Bond here, you know? It's gonna be a long few months if you look at the floor the whole time!"

I was amazed at the fact that one of the staff didn't just tell me how useless I was. It felt like a breath of fresh air. So I picked my head up and replied, "Yes, staff!"

I needed to say as few words as possible as I was really struggling to get the air into my lungs.

Surely he would leave me alone and go hassle someone else after talking to me for this long? No, he just kept staring at me, not even breathing heavily or breaking a sweat.

After another pause, he said, "Just slow your breathing down! In through the nose and out through the mouth. Slow and controlled."

He then gave me a few demonstrations and waited for me to follow suit. As soon as I was breathing as he had advised, he upped his pace and made his way to the front of the squad and left me alone.

Now this was a massive turning point for me! I went from really struggling and not being able to keep up to being one of the strongest in the squad in around a week!

This piece of advice probably changed my life. I was on the verge of failing the para selection course and being sent to my shadow posting, which was in Germany.

This piece of simple advice was like a "eureka moment" for me. It really did change the way that I trained and helped me devise a "preparation ritual" for my future training.

Since this "nudge in the right direction," I have been able to build on the advice and learned to harness it to help me, and it has helped me exponentially.

HOW TO PREPARE AND HOW TO BREATHE

First of all, let's start with the preparation. If you prepare your lungs correctly before your cardio training, you will find it a whole lot easier to get into a rhythm, you will be able to last longer on the training session, and your all-round performance and progression will be better. If you have ever started on a run, jog or fast paced walk and found that the first ten minutes are really tough because of your breathing rhythm, you will almost certainly find this piece of advice useful.

Before each and every training session, whether you are running for distance, running for time, or doing a track session, you should take the time to go through this process.

The first thing that you should do is to either sit down or stand up with your back straight and your shoulders back. Then slowly, and as deeply as you can, take a breath in through your nose until your lungs are at full capacity. Hold this for around three seconds, and then slowly exhale through your mouth until your lungs are totally empty. Then you should repeat this process for around three to five minutes.

You may think that this sounds silly, but from my experience, it is an invaluable exercise to do before any cardiovascular training.

This is something that I have done and will always do when I have any kind of cardio session ahead of me. It really does make a big difference.

If you are already a runner, you may have noticed that it takes around ten minutes to get your breathing rhythm going when you start a run. By exercising your lungs in this way, you will no longer have to go through this uncomfortable stage at the start of your cardio sessions.

BREATHING ON THE RUN

When you are actually out running, you should breathe with the same pattern that you did on the five to ten minutes preparation—in through the nose and out through the mouth, using deep controlled breaths.

At first, this may feel strange, or it may even feel that you need to breathe faster to get oxygen in quicker. It will be very tempting to abandon this slow, controlled breathing method and go for a "panic breath" type rhythm. If this does happen, I suggest that you just slow your pace down and get this breathing detail right first.

If you concentrate on feeding your body with a decent amount of oxygen, you will find your whole long-distance running experience so much better. It will become enjoyable, and you will be in a much better position to push yourself to achieve great levels of progress in a relatively short period of time.

SUMMARY

• Understand that the ability to control your breathing is a major factor when it comes to your progress and your success as a long-distance runner.

• Practice this breathing technique. You don't have to wait until your next cardio session; you can get the hang of it right now!

• Persevere with this technique and learn to keep it going throughout your cardio sessions. It may feel strange at first, but the more that you stick with it, the more that it will become second nature.

If you are really struggling on your run, you should slow your pace down and concentrate on your breathing. You can work on your pace again later. This is more important at this stage.

CHAPTER 10

WHAT TO EAT & WHEN TO EAT

Diet and nutrition is a huge and complex subject. It is probably the most complicated part of health and fitness, and you can spend years learning the ins and outs of sports-specific dietary needs.

However, if you know the basics, you can go a long way and over time build on your knowledge and trial different theories on yourself. By doing this, you will find what works best for you.

Everyone knows that food is fuel. We need this fuel to function in our everyday lives, and as a long-distance runner, you need more fuel than a "couch potato."

You don't need the right nutrition just to help you along on your training sessions; you also need to be able to fuel yourself to aid in recovery and repair.

STORY TIME

It was at the later stages of my P-company selection, and we had just finished a ten-mile session with plenty of hills thrown in. We were carrying a 35-pound backpack (not including water) and a rifle, and wearing military trousers and boots.

As the troop came to a halt after we had crossed the finish line, I noticed one of my closest friends on the course, who was standing next to me, starting to wobble. He started to pull some very strange faces before turning white and collapsing in a heap on the floor.

I quickly picked his rifle up and knelt down beside him. But before I got a chance to slap him in the face to see if I could bring him around, the staff sergeant had marched over, looking pretty angry, and was already pulling my buddy's backpack straps off.

As soon as he was out of his backpack, he was pulled to his feet and held there by the staff sergeant as he asked,

"What's your army number?" As my mate's eyes rolled back and focused on the sergeant, he reeled off his number as normal.

I was now on my feet and handed him my water. He looked at me blankly, but the staff sergeant was quick to snatch the bottle from me and force it into my buddy's hand;

"Right! What did you have for breakfast?," said the staff sergeant with a very stern tone.

"A bowl of sugar puffs," he replied quietly.

There was a short pause while the anger had a chance to boil up inside the sergeant. He then leaned right in to the still shaken and very pale recruit and blasted,

"A bowl of sugar puffs! You should know that a bowl of sugar puffs won't get you through this!"

His tone changed slightly as he backed off a bit. "You better not let this happen again. That was a stupid mistake, and at this stage of the game, you can't afford that!"

He paused again for a moment and said, "Drink up and get some scoff in you."

He then marched off to give the troop their next instruction.

As he did, I had to hold back the giggles, because all you could hear was this sergeant chuntering.

He was big, mean, and shaking his head. He looked like he was walking off to start a fight with someone, but in amongst his mumbles, I must have heard him say the phrase, "A bowl of sugar puffs," about five times.

So the moral of this story is that a bowl of sugar puffs will not get you through a hard training session!

Granted, this is not a normal situation to be in, but I'm sure that you would agree that this anecdote outlines the importance of good fuelling in the form of food for this type of training.

The number of would-be long-distance runners that only eat correctly on the day of their training surprises me. It is common practice to eat around one hour before starting your session.

But what about after your training session and all of that time you have before your next run? The time between each and every run that you go on should be used to recover and prepare yourself so you are ready to go again.

Because you are essentially training for endurance, you can afford to put in those extra calories. You are not training to be a competition bodybuilder; you are not training to look good on a beach; you are training for real function.

Don't worry if you are overweight right now. The good aesthetics will be a by-product of your efforts in long-distance running training. It will really help you to embrace this mind-set.

SO WHAT SHOULD I EAT?

Although I mentioned earlier that you don't need to be as careful as an athlete that is training for aesthetics, you do need to make sure that the calories you are consuming have a high nutrition value.

You could go to your favourite burger restaurant and consume one thousand calories from their menu, or you could stay at home and eat a more useful one thousand calories.

A very important factor in eating right for any kind of fitness training is to make sure that the calories that come from the food that you eat are high quality and nutritious.

But this section of the book is not about calorie counting; it is about choosing the right calories for your training. I want to keep it a simple as possible so it is easily actionable. I also find that you don't need to overcomplicate diet and nutrition as basic rules can be very effective.

CARBOHYDRATES

This is where you should start. Carbohydrates provide the fuel that will convert best to give you energy and longevity while running. There are simple carbohydrates that will get converted to energy right away, and there are complex carbohydrates that will give you a slower release energy source.

Your main focus when it comes to complex carbohydrates should be on getting this energy source into your body immediately after your training session and then in small amounts throughout the day and leading up to your next run.

You should make your last intake of complex carbohydrates around an hour before your training session. This time frame is just a guide, and it will vary from person to person.

If you are hungry before you start a training session, you should avoid the complex carbohydrates and focus on the simple carbohydrates. There are "energy" drinks available, but this can be a minefield. If you do go down this route, try to avoid drinks that are full of sugar. If you are stuck, go and visit a cycling shop and ask for advice.

There are all sorts of professional supplements that you can take advantage of. If you would rather stick to real food, you can eat a handful of dates, an apple, or a banana.

These types of food are very good at providing you with the energy boost that you need without causing you problems while on your run.

Your complex carbohydrate intake should be around 50% of your diet.

SUMMING UP CARBOHYDRATES

Eat complex carbs throughout the day until around an hour before your training session;

- Brown rice
- Brown pasta
- Granary bread
- Potatoes
- Oats

Eat simple carbohydrates if you need to before, during, and after your training session:

- Banana
- Apple
- Dates
- Specialist simple carb supplements

PROTEIN

Put very simply, protein is the food source that will help your body recover and repair. You need to utilise protein because the quicker that your body recovers, the quicker you will progress and the better chance you will have of staying injury-free.

Your protein intake should be around 25% of your diet. You should focus on lean forms of protein:

- Chicken breast
- Turkey
- Lean cuts of beef
- Lentils and pulses
- Quorn

• Quinoa

FATS

There is a lot of confusion over fat, so I will try not to add to this confusion. First off all, fat is not bad! In fact, you need fat in your diet to stay healthy. A good rule of thumb is that if a certain type of fat is solid at room temperature, it is not the best for you and you should probably try to avoid it. However, this is not a rule that is set in stone.

The good types of fat that you should add to your diet are:

• Avocado
• Olive oil
• Nuts (natural almonds are probably the best)
• Coconut oil
• Flax seed / Flax seed oil
• Oily fish such as salmon, sardines, and mackerel

VITAMINS AND MINERALS

You can get most of your vitamins and minerals from fruit and vegetables. A very useful rule when deciding which vegetables to add to your diet is the greener it is, the better.

Although I have listed fruits and vegetables as "vitamins and minerals," there are many other benefits to eating these, e.g., fibre content, proteins, etc. By adding this group of nutrients to your diet, you will be getting added nutritional bonuses.

Aim to eat these foods every day:

• Spinach
• Broccoli
• Cabbage
• Green beans
• Asparagus

A SAMPLE MEAL PLAN FOR A FULL DAY

It's one thing having a list of food to eat, but it's another thing actually knowing what to do with it. This is why I have added this section.

Most of the foods that have been listed here are foods that have several benefits. For example, mackerel fillets are listed in the "Fats" category. But mackerel is also a very good source of protein. So when it comes to designing your food intake plan, this is something to consider.

Here is a sample of a single day of meals for someone who is training for long distance:

Meal 1

130g (1 cup) of porridge oats with a small handful of chopped almonds
1 glass of fresh orange juice
1 banana

Meal 2

1 green leaf salad with spinach and a large mackerel fillet
1 baked potato

Meal 3

1 chicken breast
130g (1 cup) brown pasta
Green leaf salad with half an avocado
Meal 4

130g (1 cup) of porridge oats
1 scoop of high-quality whey protein powder

If you are not used to correct nutrition, this may seem like a lot of food, but if you are following the training plan outlined in the later stages of this book, or you are training in a similar way, you will need to eat this much food.

Remember that this is not only your fuel to get you through your training sessions, but it is also vital for your recovery. These sessions can put a lot of strain on you, so you need to give your body the tools that it needs to keep you at your optimum.

A FEW POINTS TO NOTE

I did not want to make this section about "calorie counting." Although calorie counts are useful to know, it is more important that you understand what food will help fuel your training and recovery in the most efficient way.

As long as you remember that it is better to have more calories than you need going in than not enough, you will be fine.

I have seen the effect of "not enough calories going in" on my own body. This was before I knew about the correct way to fuel for training.

It is almost shocking how quickly your body can become depleted if you are not eating enough during an intensive cardiovascular programme.

Make sure that you are regularly taking in water. To be fully hydrated, you will need to be constantly sipping water. It should become a habit to carry a bottle of water with you, wherever you go. This way, you can take small sips at every opportunity. This is the best way to become properly hydrated.

Before we close this chapter, I want to make a point about salt in your food. Salt can be very dehydrating, and this is something that you do not want as a long-distance runner. There are people that will disagree with me, but I would advise that you do not add salt to your meals.

CHAPTER 11

YOUR BREAD-AND-BUTTER TRAINING

"STEADY STATE"

When you eventually reach your judgment day (the day of the marathon, half marathon or personal distance goal), you will be running at a pace known as "steady state." The best way for me to explain this is:

"Running a set distance at a constant speed."

Most long-distance running events are completed at this steady-state pace. This is why it should be your "bread and butter" when it comes to your training.

If you are planning to run a long distance, maintaining a consistent pace is the best approach. By staying consistent, your body and breathing will find a rhythm, and the experience will be a whole lot more comfortable.

Although you will be running a marathon at a steady-state pace, it is not the only training method that you should utilise if you really want to succeed.

By having a strong set of lungs and a well-conditioned set of leg muscles, you will be more equipped to run these long distances.

It is for this reason that I would advise that you also throw in some interval training, hill reps, and weighted runs.

In contrast to a nice long steady-state training session, interval training and hill rep training are short bursts of fast-paced cardiovascular activity. If you include some of this type of training in the middle or at the end of your steady-state run on a weekly basis, you will be giving yourself a real edge and your progress will be that much better.

When you are comfortable with steady-state running (or roughly when you are running four to five miles as standard), you should look at introducing some hill reps, interval training, and weighted runs into your weekly routine.

Don't worry! We will cover all of these aspects and how to put it all together in other sections of this book.

If you are a beginner, you should put this out of your mind for now and focus on getting comfortable with the "steady state" side of things.

CHAPTER 12

TRAINING ON A TRACK

When I say "track training," I really mean "short bursts of max speed running" or "sprinting." For the remainder of this book, I will refer to this type of training as "track training."

Many would-be marathon/endurance runners will not even consider short bursts of track training. And in my opinion, this is a big mistake.

"If you are training for long distance, what is the use of any kind of sprint or track work?"

There are a few very good reasons to include this type of training into your running routine. First of all, it is by far the best cardiovascular workout that you can get.

If you follow the directions correctly, I am sure that you will agree with me.

First, let's look at the training that is involved; then we will cover the benefits of these sessions.

You will need:
• Your usual running kit
• A running track, football field, or large park
• A training partner or stop watch

When it comes to your "track training" day, you will get ready as usual and set off on a jog towards your track/training area. This will serve as your warm-up. If your track or training area is too far away, you can warm up once you get there.

Once you are at your track and you are ready to start training, if you haven't done so already, you should go for a steady state 15-minute jog to get you warmed up. Feel free to add a few thirty second hamstring and quad stretches.

The rest of this training session will last around twenty minutes. This does not sound like a lot, hey?

If you do this correctly, you will no doubt agree that this short session is enough to bring about effective progress.

THIS IS HOW IT WORKS:

• You sprint around your football pitch or training area of choice. It is important that this is a circuit. If you are just starting out, you can use half of the area. But be sure that your starting point is also your finishing point.

• Once you have completed your first lap, and if you have a training partner, they then immediately run the circuit. While they are running, you get to rest and recover. If you are training on your own, time your first circuit and set your stop watch to this amount of time for your rest. (Training on your own will require you to have a bit more motivation as there is no one to hold you accountable.)

• As soon as your partner gets back, it is your turn. Your rest is over! Go!

• I would suggest that you each do at least ten laps of this circuit before you stop the session.

There is no doubt that this training session will push your cardiovascular system to its limits. If you add this to your training programme, you will feel the benefits in your everyday steady-state training massively.

POINTS TO NOTE WHEN DOING YOUR TRACK TRAINING

I know that I keep stating that this is hard, but I always find that it is best to be well prepared before taking on any challenge.

If you are true to yourself and your training, you will be doing ten sprints in this session. This is you at full speed ahead!

Granted, your time around the circuit may increase each time that you complete it in your session, but you should always aim to keep each lap as close as possible time-wise to the first lap of the session. This way you are getting the most out of it.

You will probably feel sick and struggle to breathe if you have never done this type of training before. This is because your cardiovascular system (heart and lungs) is not used to this type of exertion. It is a far cry from a steady-state rhythm, and your breaths will be deeper.

To minimise this feeling, you should always try to control your breathing through the session. This does include your rest period.

You will also probably find that your legs will feel very weak and heavy. This is because your leg muscles are being pushed to new limits and trained differently to normal. It will help you out a lot if you spend some time doing quad and hamstring stretches after these sessions.

I didn't write all of this to put you off! As I said earlier, it is best to be fully aware of what to expect before you take up this challenge. It will only knock your confidence if you turn up to do the training and you can't complete it because you were not mentally or physically prepared.

We will look at how to integrate this track training into your programme in a later section of the book.

CHAPTER 13

WHAT DO YOU THINK SO FAR?

I am always eager to hear what you think of my work. I would really appreciate it if you left a review and rating on the online retail store from where you made the purchase from, and tell others about your experience.

Please take a few moments to do this if you have enjoyed this book so far.

Thanks for the feedback! ☺

CHAPTER 14

RUNNING FOR TIME

At a more advanced level of long-distance and marathon running, you may want to clear the race in a set time.

This is a further progression once you are comfortable with the distance of the course or race.

Although this may be classed as an advanced goal, it will not hurt to keep an eye on the time that it takes you to complete each run that you go on.

One of the biggest benefits of timing yourself on each run is that you will be able to work out roughly how long it takes you to cover set distances. You will know how long it takes you to run a mile, for instance.

If you keep track of this information, you will become more aware of your pace, and over time, you will be able to adjust it to set specific time goals.

In the opening chapter, I shared my own experience of timed running. After a few short weeks, I could see a marked improvement in the time it took me to cover my set distance. This then became my benchmark, and on occasion, I would set out to beat my time.

Back then, I didn't really know much about endurance and progression training. I had no one to help me, so I didn't progress as well as I could have.

I am going to suggest that you have a "test day" every two weeks. Every test day should also be a running session on a "test route."

This test route should be a route that is longer than your regular route, and every time you run your test route (it can be up to double the distance), you should try to beat the time that you previously set.

AN EXAMPLE

If your everyday route is four miles long, your test route can be up to eight miles long.

The first time that you run this, you might want to slow your pace slightly to get a feel for the extra distance. Time this run.

When the next test day comes around, try to beat this time. After your first test day, you will have a good idea of what to expect, and you will know how capable you are of the route.

If you have to stop or couldn't complete this test route, there is no need to shorten it. If you keep attempting it, with the help of your other training, you will eventually be able to beat your time week after week, and it will become more comfortable.

I would strongly urge you not to give up on this route. If you have to walk, you have to walk. No big deal. But it is important that each time that you attempt it, you note down the time that it took you.

CHAPTER 15

RUNNING FOR DISTANCE

The big question is,

"Can I run twenty-six miles in one shot?"

It is unlikely that your body will let you do this without the correct conditioning. And it would not pay off well to just start training with huge distances like this.

Of course you will have doubts about your ability to run this kind of distance, but with the right training structure, mind-set, and body conditioning, you can develop a great tolerance to the stress that this causes on your body.

There is no denying that twenty-six miles is a big distance and it will put your body under a huge amount of stress, but the fitter that you are endurance-wise, the easier that you will be able to deal with this.

The recovery time after a twenty-six mile run is probably the best part of a week or longer, depending on the individual.

It is for this reason that you should not run these kinds of distances on a regular basis. If you do, you will no doubt have to quit due to injury sooner rather than later.

Instead of using "distance per running session" as your main measure of progression, I would suggest that you use "distance run per week." This is a great way to see that you are heading in the right direction. And the more miles that you clock up, the better equipped you will be physically and mentally for your race day.

As you will soon see in the Putting It All Together section, I have outlined set distances for you to run each training session. These progress on a weekly basis, starting at two miles per session and increasing to seven.

You may be thinking that seven miles is nothing compared to twenty-six, but the other elements in your training routine will compliment this to condition you so you are more than ready for race day.

So keep in mind that your distance per session is not the deciding factor when it comes to your ability to be able to run a marathon.

CHAPTER 16

RUNNING WITH WEIGHT

A weighted backpack can be a very effective tool for long-distance running and endurance. Although this idea is shunned by a lot of people, if you think about it logically, it's a no-brainer.

Look at it this way; if you were to run a ten-mile route every day for thirty days wearing a weighted backpack and then you ran the same route on the thirty-first day without the backpack, what do you think your run on the thirty-first day would be like?

It would be like a breath of fresh air. You would have no problem getting around this route, and you may even be able to do an extra few miles in the same amount of time. You may also find that you can comfortably up your pace and push yourself to another level.

As you can see, I am "pro" wearing a weighted backpack when it comes to endurance training. Because, after all, if you are a good endurance runner, you are a good marathon runner.

HOW TO PACK YOUR BACKPACK
Putting some bricks or dumbbells in a backpack is all well and good in theory, but in practice, it's a whole different story.

It's no good just filling a backpack with any old heavy objects that you can lay your hands on, and it's no good just using any old backpack that you can find.

Although running with weight is a great way to improve your endurance, a badly selected, badly fitted, and badly packed backpack can cause you all sorts of problems from back injury to severe chafing.

These things can really hinder your training. This is why you should never go into weighted running lightly. You should take a bit of advice from someone that knows the score.

First off, let's look at the type of backpack that you should invest in.

Before rushing out and buying the cheapest backpack, it is worth understanding that comfort and stability are a must if you are to utilise this tool as part of your training. This backpack will be used a lot and will become one of your "running buddies."

DURABILITY

The harder wearing that your backpack is, the better. Rigid hard-wearing material will last you longer and it is less likely to deteriorate when exposed to harsh weather conditions and extended use.

FITTING

Your new backpack should have two identical shoulder straps that are well padded and adjustable. It should have a large surface area that is in contact with your back during use. This part of your backpack should also have a certain amount of padding. An optional extra is a padded waist support.

FUNCTIONALITY

It should have "top opening," meaning that anything that you put into the backpack goes in through the top. It should have a top opening flap as access to the main compartment that can be adjusted when closed rather than a zip. The backpack's container compartment should ideally be rectangular and symmetrical.

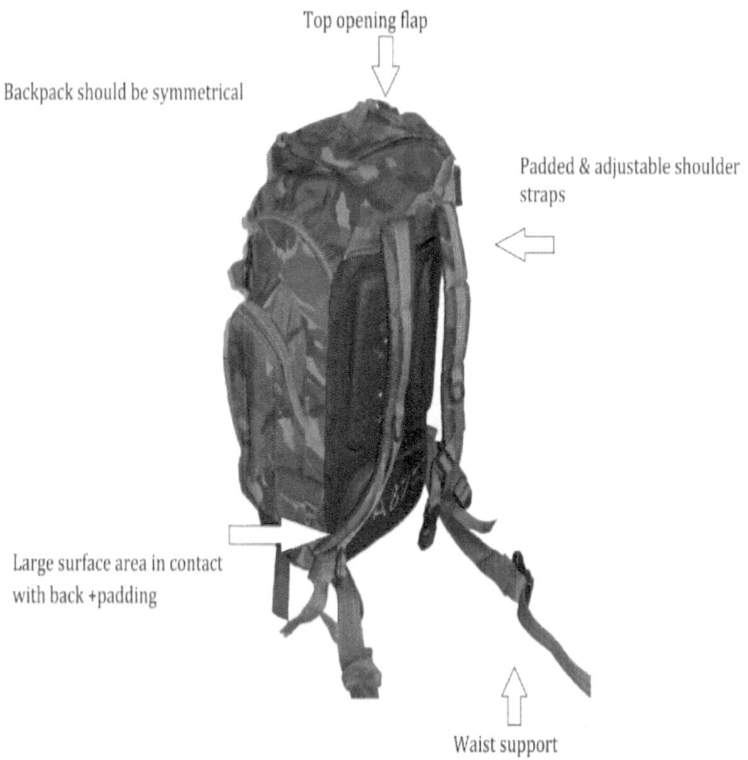

Now that you have a decent backpack, it's time to get it set up for your weighted runs!

It is unlikely that you'll set up your weighted backpack to your liking on your very first weighted run. Although I hope you do, the reality is that you will need to tweak, tighten, and shift the position of the straps and the contents of the backpack to get it just right.

Hopefully, this guide will save you a whole lot of guesswork, pain, and frustration and put you on the right track.

ADDING YOUR WEIGHT

When packing a Burgan for a ten- or twenty-mile tab in my old squadron, the weight used had to be "useful kit," so we couldn't use a big bag of sand or something along those lines. We had to use items that we would normally use for our job, and we had to find 38 pounds worth of this.

In our case now, though, we can use anything that we want! I would

suggest deciding how much weight you want to start with and
getting this in the form of a bag of sand.

Sand is great for this, as it can be moulded and evenly distributed. Also, by using sand instead of something like dumbbell plates or bricks, you will have no sharp bits that have the potential to shift mid run and stick in your back.

Let's say that you have now got a ten-pound bag of sand. (This is the weight that I suggest that you start with; you can always add more later.) You now need to pack this into your backpack correctly.

If you are packing a weighted backpack with a bag of sand or any other deadweight for that matter, it is very important to put this weight right at the top. It was a while into my training that I learned this.

If you have the heaviest part of your backpack closest to your head, you will benefit in several ways. First and probably most important, the weight that is high on your back will pull your shoulders backwards, helping you to keep good posture and opening up your lungs when running.

If you have the weight right at the bottom of your backpack, it will be resting on the small of your back and you will have a tendency to lean forward when running. This is not good, and it would not be long before you were suffering from back pain.

A more practical reason for having the weight at the top of your backpack is that if it moves to an "unbalanced" position during your run, you can easily access it and sort it out.

So how do you get ten pounds of sand at the top of your backpack without filling your backpack first?

Well, you fill your backpack first! The best way to do this is to find pillows, cushions, or bulky clothing items that you no longer use. The weight from these will be negligible.

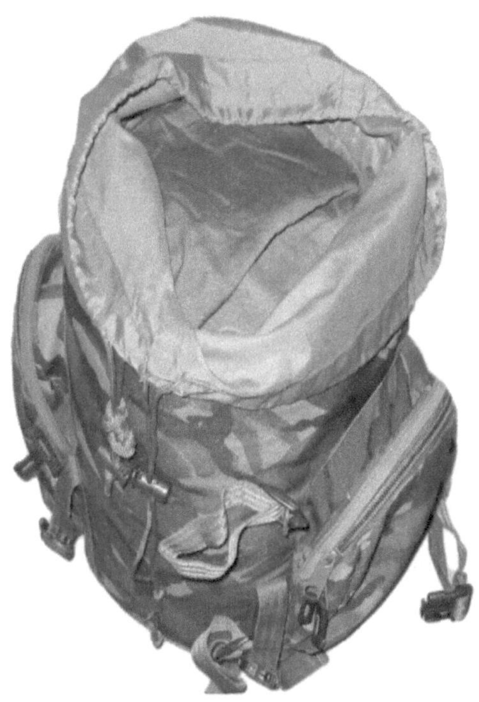

Backpack has been packed out with bulky soft clothing

It is a good idea to waterproof these before you put them into your backpack. Put them in bin bags, or if you feel like pushing the boat out, you can get a backpack liner or canoe bag. Remember—when stuffing your pack with your base filling, you should consider symmetry and even distribution.

When you have filled your backpack to the top, you can then add your weight.

As mentioned earlier, sand can be moulded. This is great because it will allow you to pack your backpack with an even weight distribution.

After you have your bag of sand, you should fashion this into some kind of tight symmetrical shape.

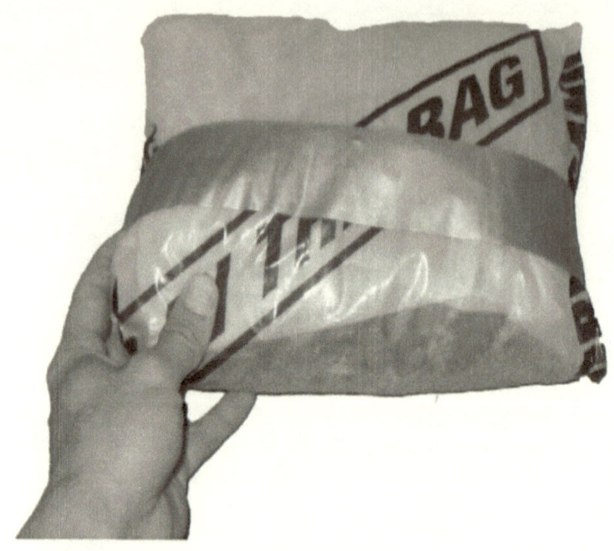

I've seen plenty of these on crime shows... but this is just a bunch of gravel.

If your weight is in a form that resembles this, you can then place the package at the very top and centre of your backpack.

Once that this is in, you may want to add a bit more in the way of bulky light material to secure the weight in place. When you are happy, close your backpack and tighten it up using the adjustable top flap.

The last thing that you need to do in the packing of your backpack is make it as solid a unit as possible. If anything in the backpack (including the weight) moves when you pick it up and shake it slightly, you have not packed it tightly enough.

Go back and add more "stuffing" under the sand. If you have a backpack that opens from the top with adjustable straps, you can pull these tighter and this should solve the problem.

It can be really annoying to have excess straps flying around when you are running with a backpack on, so feel free to fold these up and tape them.

Here is my finished backpack: solid, symmetrical and with evenly distributed weight. It is now ready to be fitted and adjusted.

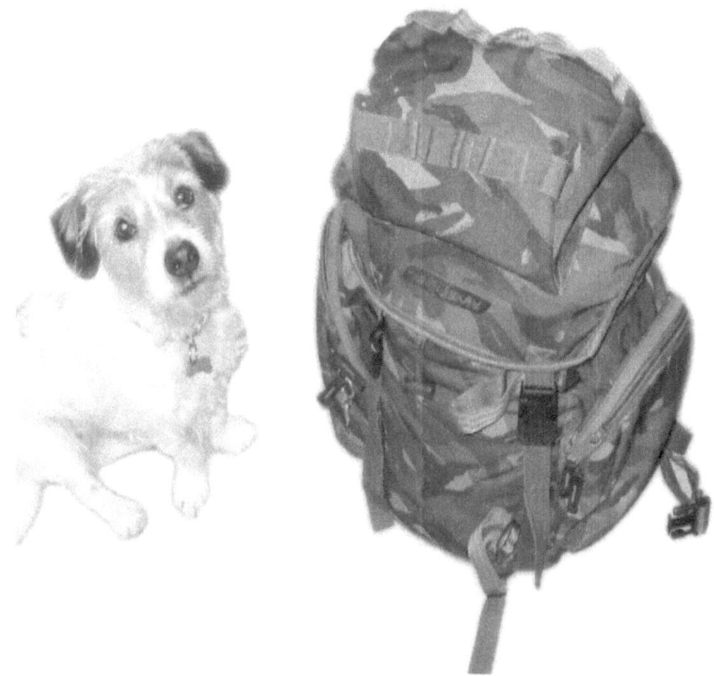

Packed backpack, approved by my little buddy

FITTING YOUR WEIGHTED BACKPACK

When you first put your backpack on, you should feel the benefit of putting the weight at the top. The pack should pull your shoulders back slightly and not force you to stoop forward.

The weight of your pack should feel evenly distributed, and you should have no points of discomfort in the way of sharp objects pressing against your back. If you do feel anything—maybe a button from an item of clothing has been packed tightly and you can feel this slightly on your back—you should sort this out.

Even a small thing like this can cause you problems when out on your run. It is surprising what damage something as small as this can do in the way of chafing.

At the final fitting, your backpack should;

• Be a solid unit with even weight distribution

• Have the weight secured in the top, also evenly distributed

• Be free of uncomfortable points when rested on your back

• Stay tight to your back when running. If it does not, you should tighten the straps and/or utilise the waist strap.

CHAPTER 17

DEALING WITH BLISTERS AND CHAFING

Staying free of blisters and chafing is a must if you plan to progress in your marathon training.

Fortunately, there are a lot of products that you can try to prevent this type of thing. Products ranging from topical creams and plasters to inner soles are all readily available for you to try out.

The problem is that there are just too many products for you to test. I have been in this situation before, and I make no illusions as to the impact on your training that blisters and chafing can have.

Back when I did the "beat up course" for para training, one of the guys on the course decided to buy some "anti-shock," "anti-blister" inner soles for his boots. He had seen an advert somewhere that claimed these inner soles would really help to protect his knees from the constant shock of running and also reduce the chance of blisters.

Wanting to stay free of these common injuries, he spent upwards of £20 on these inner soles, fitted them into his boots, and started on what would be his last training session with the airborne forces.

During the long training session, he struggled a fair bit, but due to the nature of the training, he didn't really get any sympathy—he just pushed through it.

By the time we had finished and he eventually got to take his boots off, the blisters had developed and popped, and his socks were stained with blood. This is the worst case of blisters that I have ever seen.

It took a week before this guy could even wear socks again. The rubbing that had caused these pretty shocking injuries had cost him his career with airborne forces. Because of this injury, he fell back with the training progress and was forced to return to his unit in Germany. I never saw him again.

I will always remember this incident, and I have learned a lot from someone else's mistakes. It was probably down to this guy's mistakes that I learned to take good care of my own feet.

If I had not seen firsthand that a small change such as "helpful inner soles" could be so devastating, I would have probably tried this type of thing myself.

Needless to say, I stuck to the advice of one of the more experienced para training staff. This advice ensured that I did not get any blisters that hindered my progress, and subsequently, I went on to pass the course!

"Jim! Stop telling stories and tell me how you avoid getting blisters already!" I hear you say.

Okay, this is how I stay blister free, and hand on heart, I swear by it!

Wear two pairs of socks! Simple.

Well there's a bit more to it than that, but that's the basic secret.

If you think about it, this does make a lot of sense. Blisters are caused by friction from constant movement in a very localised area.

With this constant friction on your heel, toes, or any other part of your foot, your body reacts.

Fluid forms between the upper layers of the affected skin in an attempt to cushion and heal the area, but if the rubbing continues, this will burst and the process may start again on the new layers of skin. If the rubbing still continues, it will run out of skin to protect, and this will be extremely painful.

So all you have to do is stop the rubbing. If you put on a thin and fairly tight pair of cotton socks and then put a pair of hiking type socks on over these, any rubbing from your footwear will not affect your feet because the energy will be between the pairs of socks.

There are no fancy products or lotions, just a very simple logical and effective solution!

After I started using this method, the only area of slight discomfort and potential for blister development was where my toes would rub against each other. This was easily solved by just wrapping the affected toe with a single layer of medical tape.

We used to run every day, and if we were not running in boots, I would not need to use this tape; the two pairs of socks were more than enough.

One last thing: although it may be common sense to many, I think it is worth mentioning, as it took me a blister or two to figure it out. If you have running shoes that have laces, you should never tuck the excess lace from the bow you tie into your shoes. Even if you are wearing two pairs of socks and have medical tape all over your feet, this can still cause you hot spots or blisters and be very uncomfortable.

I have always run in training shoes with laces, and if the laces are too long, I will simply cut them down and burn the ends to stop any fraying. This is worth doing if you are in the same boat.

CHAFING IN OTHER AREAS

Luckily for me, I never suffered from any other type of chafing but unfortunately have seen my fair share of others who have.

First, I want to cover (no pun intended) "nipple chafing." This is a very common problem for long-distance runners.

This is more of a problem for male runners, as the nipples are normally in direct contact with the outer layer of clothing.

The small, constant movements of the outer layer of clothing can cause the area around the nipples to become very sore.

You can put two small strips of medical tape in a sort of "cross" formation over each nipple, and this will stop the irritation.

I have heard of people just using a petroleum based gel, but in my experience, this is nowhere near as effective as the tape.

Another option is to invest in a tightly fitting running top. Something like an Under Armour base layer is a good choice.

Another area that can be affected by chafing is the upper inner thigh. I have never really had a problem with this, but I know plenty of people who have.

If you suffer from this problem, you could first get yourself some tight cycling shorts to wear underneath your regular running bottoms. Like we mentioned earlier, this will put another layer between the rubbing effects and take away the chance of irritation.

Personally, I think that this is the best solution, but I understand that some people find these uncomfortable to wear.

You could also try a bit of Vaseline, but this may wear off. Another way to try and avoid this type of chafing is to use an antiperspirant spray.

This will reduce any sweating and also put a small barrier of powder on the area. I have not seen this done to good effect, but it is something you may want to try.

CHAPTER 18

STAYING INJURY-FREE

It is very important that you stay as injury-free as possible. Any type of niggle or awkward pain can cause you big problems. If you do have pain in a localised part of your body after a run or training session, you should address this right away.

The first thing that you should do is use an ice pack on the area. This will help to control any inflammation. If the pain gets worse after resting or during future training sessions, you should immediately see your physician.

If you get reoccurring pain in a certain area, you should try to work out what is causing this. It may be your running style; check that your running position is as per the checklist in this book, and check that your running shoes are serviceable and they are of good quality.

If you do start to feel any pain, you should not ignore it! Ignoring a possible injury will only make it worse, and you will run the risk of not being able to train at all. You could even end up back at square one or worse!

So please take care of yourself. If you feel pain:

Rest
Ice
Compression
Elevation

Remember "RICE".

I learned this acronym when I first joined the army. It is used for strains and pulled muscles, but it will pay to use this on any muscular discomfort.

I also learned that the more vigilant you are with these aches and pains, the better health you will be in and the further you will get.

So it will pay off to take extra care when it comes to the well-being of your body. Remember that long-distance running will put you and your body under a lot of stress.

CHAPTER 19

IT'S ALL IN THE MIND

There is a lot to be said about the power of the mind and mental robustness. This is a trait and indeed an aspect of training and fitness progression that I have learned to regard as one of the most valuable and priceless qualities that you can work to develop.

Doubts and self-limitation are products of your own mind and can drastically hold you back from achieving any goal.

As mentioned throughout this book, a British airborne soldier can only call themselves such if they pass the rigors of P company and to do this, he must have already, or learn to have a mind that will never give up.

While I was serving with 9 squadron, there were a fair few events put on to encourage the whole brigade to interact with each other. This meant that there would be military engineers from all different areas of the army in one place. These events were always set up to be physically competitive.

One such event was put on just before we were due to go on summer leave one year. This was a big event that was hosted over two days at a well-equipped training area. I can't remember exactly where as this didn't really matter at the time. All I knew was that this was a competition that involved all of the squadrons that were attached to the brigade and more. So it was a big event.

The nature of this sporting event was that there were a handful of physical activities that had an element of competition to them. To name a few of these, there was a rowing machine race, a rugby sevens tournament, a soccer tournament, a five man team assault course, some kind of sprint event and the last event was a ten mile cross country running race.

Everyone could only pick two events to compete in with the exception of the cross country running event which everyone could choose to do to try and get extra points for their squadron.

The cross country running race was the last event as it was the biggest. All of the squadrons involved in this event put forward their best long distance runners, all apart from my squadron who put forward all of their squadron to a man. This was because every member of 9 squadron was capable of running ten miles and the rules of the competition allowed no limit to the amount of runners in this event.

As this was a big event we were split up into smaller groups, groups of about thirty and set off at staggered timings to minimise bottle necks and crowding. It all started as you would expect, the stronger runners shot ahead, and it was clear to me that there were some very competent runners from other "none airborne" squadrons that had more than a good chance of winning this race or coming in with completive run times.

As I and every other 9 squadron bloke here were used to running on all types of terrain and elevation variants, it was like any other "day at the office". I always got the feeling that other squadrons in the engineers looked at us with a kind of reluctant respect. I will admit that there was a lot of arrogance that came from many who wore a maroon beret or maroon t-shirt with embroidered para wings stitched on the chest, so there were plenty of runners here from regular squadrons that would love to beat a 9 squadron guy in this race.

Everyone from the regular engineer units would wear green t-shirts, but the 9 squadron guys wore maroon, so we stuck out and you could see us coming. We were about eight miles into the race and as you can imagine, we were all spread out across several miles by now. I remember this course being fairly easy and found myself passing a lot of other runners.

At around this eight mile mark, I was gaining on a non 9 squadron guy (a green t-shirt), he must have been about one hundred meters in front of me and I noticed him make an over the shoulder glance to see if anyone was behind him, and I knew right away that he saw the maroon t-shirt that I was wearing. As we only had about two miles to go, he just needed to keep this distance between me and him and he would have beaten a 9 squadron guy in a running race. He upped his pace and I found that the gap between me and him was no longer closing. He was a fair distance in front of me and I noticed that he kept glancing around to see that I wasn't gaining on him.

He really wanted to beat me but I didn't really want to get beaten by a "normal" cross country runner or a green t-shirt, so I upped my pace also. We ran like this for about a mile maintaining this on hundred meter gap. He would still glance around every now and again to make sure I wasn't getting any closer.

As we were near the end of the race, I decided to up my pace a bit more and started to close the gap. Right away he noticed this and upped his pace also. When he did this I would up my pace again and again and every time he turned around to see how far away I was, I would be a bit closer to him until eventually, I was about ten meters away. At this point when he turned to glance over his shoulder, he gave me an exasperated smile and let me pass, admitting defeat. Although I was confident that I was going to beat him, I was glad that he decided to give up because it made things easier for me. I was expected to win because of the colour that I was wearing.

I often think of this situation and the impact that the mind can have on people. I also wonder if the one variable that kept me confident and gave him doubt was removed, would he have given up at all?

This guy that I was running against was a formidable runner and was chosen to run for his squadron. He was doing well in this race and I believe that his fitness levels were above average, he was built for cross country running and maybe if he had not doubted himself, he would have been able to beat me.

The very thing that gave me the confidence to push him to defeat was the thing that made him doubt himself. I am 90% sure that if I wasn't wearing that maroon t-shirt, it might have been a different story. From my point of view; I am expected to win, I am wearing the maroon of an airborne soldier, I am a machine and cannot be beaten. From his point of view; he is competing against someone one who is wearing a maroon t shirt, someone from 9 squadron, this is a guy that will not quit, he is a machine that can't be beaten.

Looking back at it, it amazes me how a simple colour and what it represents can change the mind-set of someone. If I was wearing a regular green t-shirt, maybe I would not be as confident to push to beat him and maybe he would have had the confidence to keep going and not let me pass.

This is a lesson that always pops into my head when I see people walking on their running sessions or see people giving up before they really have to. In my experience, it is very rare that someone will stop when they are actually exhausted or at their physical limits and it is more likely that they will stop when their mind tells them to.

I am not saying that every training session should bring you to physical exhaustion but you should test yourself and find your limits because this will tell you how fit you really are, in body and mind, and wat you now believe to be your physical limits may be very far away from the reality. If this is the case, you may find progression very slow or find it really hard to get any results at all when it comes to your running and fitness goals.

CHAPTER 20

FIND SOME MOTIVATORS

Staying motivated is a tricky business and the simplicity of self-motivation varies for everyone. Luckily, if you are someone who struggles with motivation when it comes to training sessions, I have a few tips that you might like to try if you do not do so already. Here are four tips that you can try to keep you motivated:

Tip one – Motivational quotes

In a few of my other books, I recommend creating a bunch of motivational quotes that you can personalise and put around your life. This is something that I have done in the past and still do now. I use this motivation tactic to help me with more than just my fitness goals, I use it for my business plans, and even my writing and publishing goals.

It has been very valuable to me and I'm really glad that I gave it a chance as when I started doing this I did it with more than a bit of scepticism.

If you are willing to give this a try, all you need to do is to think about why you want to hit your running goals (or other goals that you might want to use this for) and write these down. You can even search the internet for good fitness motivational quotes and you will find some great, ready-made ones.

I suggest that you find at least five of these. When you have these, you should make them look eye-catching. By this, I mean that they should be big and bold. You should not have to squint to read them when they are in eye shot, I find that an A5 paper size is a good benchmark and they should be colourful where possible.

Once you have your motivational quotes, you should pin them up. But you should put them were you will see them more than once per day. It is a good idea to have these where you spend most of your time so they will always be in your face to remind you why you are doing what you are doing and why you have set your goals.

Tip Two – Listen to music, podcasts or audio books

For me, running sessions, bike journeys and any form of cardio for that matter mean music. Sometimes I will decide to go for a run or do a cardio session for an excuse to listen to some music or a certain playlist that I have created.

Not only does music get me up off the sofa and out of the door, but when I am actually doing the cardio work, it spurs me on and sometimes inspires me to challenge myself more and push myself that bit harder.

I have a fairly diverse range when it comes to music taste but Metallica, Iron maiden and music from people like Brian Fallon are a big part of my running playlists. This is the type of music that inspires me but I know that different things provoke different responses in different people. For instance, I know that Matt, the narrator of my audio books likes to listen to 80s rock ballads or the Rocky sound track when he is doing cardio sessions, but in his Pilates sessions, he likes to listen to the spice girls and the like. ☺

If you are not a fan of music, you may have other interests or hobbies. There is no better time to learn about new things, develop your knowledge of a subject that you are interested in, catch up on news or listen to a novel or series of novels than during your running sessions. These days, it is becoming increasingly easier to access information on any subject through audio books and podcasts, so if you have an interest that you wouldn't mind learning more about, just get a play list of this sorted, download a bunch of interesting podcasts or audio books and get them on a playlist. The more the merrier!

If you are new to running or you find cardio boring and mundane and you haven't tried music, podcasts, audio novels, audio dramas, informational products, or you have become complacent with your choice of audio, it may be a good idea to experiment with a few different options. Don't underestimate how motivating this could be.

Tip 3 – Get a running app or GPS tracker

When I first started running, there was no such thing as a running app. This was before smart phones and android devices were available. Although most of my friends and family will tell you that I still don't know what to do with a mobile phone, I can assure you that I have found great motivation from a running app or two.

There are plenty of running apps that can be downloaded to your smart phone, but the one that I use is called "Strava". I am not affiliated with these guys but I will recommend this app as I have had good experiences with it and still use it today.

What does a running app have to do with motivation? Well I can tell you that from the first run that I set out on whilst using my new app, I was motivated by the results. This type of motivation wasn't as obvious as my favourite music being pumped into my ears or the thought of a powerful reason that pushed me forward to achieve my goals bought on by a motivational quote. This was a bit more subtle. When I had finished my first run, I found that I could see how many miles that I had run, I could see a map display with a red line that represented the route that I had covered and I could see the time that it had taken me. This was real-time tracking and the data was saved for me to look back on. It's great because this information can be used for visual progression.

The motivator that is most valuable for me from this app is the "weekly" statistic. Among other things, the weekly statistic tells you how many miles are covered. It's a really good feeling to say, "this week I ran thirty five miles"

Since I stepped into the modern world (I'm always slow off the mark but after all – "Slow and steady wins the race") and got myself familiar with a running app, this app has become like my music when it comes to my cardio sessions. It has actually become the reason that my phone is now always charged and with me…. Most of the time.

So if you are also slow off the mark and have not embraced running apps, you should definitely look into this. The one that I have mentioned is one of many and I know that there are dedicated devices that track more data than distance travelled and time passed. So it might be worth investing in one of these. After all, you might find that keeping track of something more personal like watching your resting heart rate drop from week to week will be a big motivator. This is an example of data that can be tracked with a more dedicated piece of kit.

Tip 4 – Make a physical wall chart

This is another one of my favourite motivators that not only works for running motivation but it also works for all kinds of other fitness goals.

It's all well and good having a GPS tracker or running app on your mobile device and keeping track of your progress and motivation this way, but when all is said and done, this data and motivator is hidden away in its app and only deciding to appear when you ask it to.

If you have a dedicated physical wall chart that uses the old "mark one" pen and paper to record this, you are committing to a little bit more in my opinion.

This is how I would play it – I would take some time to create a simple chart that displays weeks, days and months in the headers or take advantage of a shop bought calendar if you struggle to get your head around a personal creation. Once you have this, you can plan your training sessions in advance and tick them off as you go. When you complete one of your planned training sessions, you can tick it off with a bright happy colour. When you miss one of your training sessions you can put a cross through it with a dark colour. You will want to see bright ticks over your training plan, not dark crosses. This is a great motivator in my experience.

I love to use physical wall charts to monitor my progress and keep me motivated. The unique trait that a wall chart offers is that it doesn't hide away, it doesn't lie and it will be brutally honest with you when it comes to checking your progress.

Staying motivated can be hard work and as a passionate fitness instructor, writer and general all round health and fitness enthusiast myself, it always saddens me to see the fitness potential of an individual go to waste due to a lack of motivation. If you are someone who really struggles with motivation, you should make it a priority to learn how to self-motivate. This is a skill that is generally overlooked but once you figure it out, it offers huge rewards. A good start would be to pick one, or all of the above motivators and work towards putting them into practice. You may be surprised how much these ideas help if you have not dabbled in them before.

If you would like more information on the development of fitness and exercise motivation, I have taken care of this in one of my other books. It is appropriately titled – "Fitness & Exercise Motivation" by James Atkinson and it is also available in audio format so you can even listen while you run.

CHAPTER 21

YOUR PROGRESSION IS RELATIVE TO YOUR TRAINING

Most people know the age old theory that tells; if you put a small fish into a small tank, the fish won't grow, if you put the small fish into a large tank, it will grow a whole lot bigger. This basically means that a fish will grow to the size of its tank.

The same goes for training progression. A lot of people are guilty of falling into a routine with no progression. This is great if you are not looking to progress in your chosen fitness niche, and just want to maintain a healthy lifestyle or you are happy with the fitness level that you have. Kudos to this group of people. But if you do want to change, and progress with your running or any aspect of your fitness for that matter, you have to challenging yourself when you reach new heights. Or, metaphorically, you have to get yourself a bigger tank to live in, as the proverb states.

I was recently reminded of this lesson during my own fitness endeavours. I have biked to the gym and back for the last four years. This six mile round trip (split in half by a weight training session when I actually arrived at the gym) has remained a challenge for this duration, and I am sure that you will agree that four years is a long time to struggle with anything.

There were many times that I questioned my fitness levels and made excuses for this challenging part of my training in this time, and there were more than a few times when I thought that there was something wrong with me because these two short stints of three miles would sometimes leave me totally exhausted. Of course, there was always the assumption that I was struggling so much because of the hard resistance training that I would do when I was actually in the gym, this was a very plausible explanation for my challenging bike rides that sandwiched this "resistance training" priority of mine.

You would think that after this amount of time, cycling to the gym would become like second nature and it would become effortless. But no, it never got any easier and remained a challenge, until I changed a few things, nearly by accident.

When I first decided to become a fitness author, I gave up my car. How can an unknown fitness author with no publisher and moreover, not a single book to his name afford to run a car? I had an old bike at this point and decided that this would be my main mode of transport. Fast forward several years; I now have several books to my name and I am making a living and am in a position where I am able to invest in a car again, like a "normal person".

In the time I have been without a car and have been using a push bike as my main mode of transport, this has forged my habits and lifestyle into something that I have come to enjoy. I also appreciate the extra health benefits that cycling is responsible for, and I don't want to give that up. So instead of buying a car, I decided to invest in a brand new, quality push bike.

In the time that I have been using a bike as my main mode of transport, I have only ever had "hand me downs" or very cheap options. But now I have a higher standard of bike, its much nicer to ride.

However, when I first started riding this to the gym as I would normally do, it was still just as challenging physically. But because I had this new comfortable bike, I decided to start biking to my parents' house that was about ten miles away. I started doing this about twice per week when I had a "rest day" in my gym training schedule. On these days, I would pack my laptop into its back pack, throw it on my back, and head off on the ten miler to work from my parents' house for the day. It's always nice to have a change of scenery in your working life from time to time.

Although I struggled a bit at first with this big jump to ten miles in one session as opposed to the three that I had been used to, after a few short weeks of doing these supplemental bike rides, I noticed that on my training days, the journey to and from the gym became significantly easier. In fact, I would go as far as saying that my journey to the gym has become easy! So in essence, four years of struggling has been remedied by a relatively small change over several weeks. This is pretty amazing when you think about it.

Although I can reel off stories and anecdotes about my past running achievements to highlight this point, I thought that it would be nice to demonstrate this fundamental element of fitness training through my more recent training activities whilst also pointing out that progression is extremely important in all areas of fitness, not just running and other cardio activities.

When it comes to running, you have to take training progression into consideration. The simple training routine that I have suggested in this book has a progressive characteristic at its core and I would advise that even if you decided not to follow a single part of this routine, that you at least follow a routine that does have a progressive nature, and when you hit your goal, if you would like to make a more lofty goal, that you tweak your training accordingly.

If a Marathon runner decided that he or she wanted to continue to be a long distance runner but only wanted to train by doing a slow, three mile jog once per week from now on. A or month or two later, they would really struggle and eventually no longer be able to run a marathon. If the same runner decided that they would like to up their game, and become an ultra-marathon runner, they would have to adjust their training accordingly and go through the struggle of reaching the next goal. In time, this runner would be able to breeze through a single marathon with less effort than they had ever expended before.

Going back to your training now; If you would like the next six months of fitness progression to be like the last six months, keep doing what you are doing. But if you are not happy with the way your training is going, you need to look at making some changes. Everyone is different and some are slower to develop than others, but it is always worth challenging yourself and removing yourself from that comfort zone if you truly want to progress.

When I first started running, I ran a timed, two mile circuit every day in order to pass the standard one and a half mile fitness test for entry into the army. This was my goal and had that been my ultimate running goal, I would have never changed my running style, my running speed or the distance that I ran. My body would never have been challenged any more than this, so I would have effectively lived in the same small tank that the small fish lived in. Granted, this tank would be bigger than other fishes but I would always have the option to move to a bigger tank. Hopefully I have demonstrated in this book how this metaphor has been apparent, not just in my running progress but in my entire fitness journey.

So if you really want to make progress and become better than you are at what you do, you have to grow and get yourself out of your comfort zone, challenge yourself more than you have previously done so and you will continue to grow and develop. A good measure of your progress is to try something that you used to find challenging (let's say a running route that you used to struggle on) and if this is far from the struggle that you remember, you are on the right track.

If you continue to progress, your toughest challenges right now will eventually turn into "a trip down easy street".

CHAPTER 22

PUTTING IT ALL TOGETHER (YOUR TRAINING PLAN)

In this section, I will outline a solid progressive training plan. You can follow this exactly or you can use parts of this to add to another training plan or create your own.

You will notice that we are utilising the training methods that have been mentioned in earlier chapters of this book. So if you just skipped to this section, it might not make much sense.

The training plan is set out on a twelve-week time frame. But I am very aware that some people will develop and progress more quickly than others. So if you reach a week that you really struggle with, just repeat it until you are ready to move on.

I will say that if you do want progress, you should always push yourself to the next level. So please don't fall into the trap of staying on a certain week for months on end, because your fitness progression will soon become stagnant.

ADDING YOUR WEIGHT, OPTIONAL BUT ADVISED

This is up to you; you can add your weighted backpack to your training at any point. I would suggest that if you are going to add this to your running sessions that you do it in the early stages. Once you start with this weight, you should always run with it, with the exception of "track day" training, unless you are planning to get "superman" fit. If you get used to running with the extra weight as standard, you will find any training session or your marathon a lot easier.

POINTS TO NOTE

Please take some time to look over the different training weeks before you start. You will notice that the workload on the last few weeks of this programme lightens up.

This is because in the last few weeks that lead up to the race, your body will need to be running at its optimum performance and be fully recovered.

It may feel strange to "slack off" at this point, but you must be responsible. It would be a shame to get this far just to struggle more than you need to on race day.

Remember; you have done all of the hard work already, and it is time to recuperate and be at the top of your game when it comes to your big day.

You will also notice that at around the halfway point in this programme, there is an easy week or two. This is because it is good to take your foot off the gas slightly at fairly regular intervals in order to aid recovery and prevent injury in a training programme like this one.

Week 1
3 x 2 miles per training day
1 x track day - (See the "training on a track chapter 12")
Rest 2 days
Test day (Friday): 3 miles
9 miles this week (not including track day)

Week 2
3 x 3 miles per training day
1 x track day - (See the "training on a track chapter")
Rest 2 days
Test day (Friday): 4 miles
13 miles this week (not including track day)

Week 3
3 x 4 miles per training day
1 x track day - (See the "training on a track chapter")
Rest 2 days
Test day (Friday): 5 miles
17 miles this week (not including track day)

Week 4
3 x 5 miles per training day
1 x track day - (See the "training on a track chapter")
Rest 2 days
Test day (Friday): 6 miles
21 miles this week (not including track day)

Week 5
3 x 6 miles per training day
1 x track day - (See the "training on a track chapter")
Rest 2 days
Test day (Friday): 7 miles
25 miles this week (not including track day)

Week 6
2 x 7 mile per training day
No track day
Rest 3 days
Test day (Friday): 8 miles
22 miles this week (not including track day)

Week 7
3 x 6 miles per training day
1 x track day - (See the "training on a track chapter")
Rest 2 days
Test day (Friday): 7 miles
25 miles this week (not including track day)

Week 8
3 x 6 miles per training day
1 x track day - (See the "training on a track chapter")
Rest 2 days
Test day (Friday): 10 miles
28 miles this week (not including track day)

Week 9
3 x 5 miles per training day
1 x track day - (See the "training on a track chapter")
Rest 3 days
Test day (Friday): 10 miles
25 miles this week (not including track day)

Week 10
3 x 5 miles per training day
No track day
Rest 3 days

Test day (Friday): 12 miles
27 miles this week

Week 11
3 x 5 miles per training day
No track day
Rest 3 days
Test day (Friday): 15 miles
30 miles this week

Week 12
3 x 5 miles per training day
No track day
Rest 4 days
No test day
15 miles this week

CHAPTER 23

RACE DAY!

If you have decided to go ahead and run a half or full Marathon, there are a few things that I think are worth considering before the day, and actually on the day of the race. Some of the following tips may seem simple but in my experience of long distance running, I have made these mistakes more than once, and it would be a shame to ruin your race day by making a trivial error. Here are some points to note to ensure that you are suitably prepared.

On the week that leads up to your race day, you should be doing minimal exercise. As mentioned earlier, you have done the hard work at this point, and you are ready whether you believe it or not.

I would advise that you do not do any running at all for about four days before the race; you should continue to eat as you did throughout your training until the day before. In the last twenty-four hours, you should do nothing at all: sit around, watch TV, play computer games, and stay off your feet as much as possible.

It is common knowledge to "carb load" also in this last twenty-four hours. The food that you put into your body at this stage will be the fuel that your body uses for your big day.

While you are sitting around, you should have an endless supply of water on hand and be sipping on this constantly.

You should have plenty of brown pasta, brown rice, and plenty of protein on hand.

A lot of people will advise you to just cram it in until you feel bloated, then cram in some more. But I believe that this will just make you feel uncomfortable.

Try eating one cup of high-quality, slow-release carbohydrates every two hours. You should also be adding a lot of good fats and protein to each of these meals.

Remember to look after your feet; make sure that they are clean and your toenails are trimmed.

Prep your kit; make sure that you have whatever "blister repellent" has served you well in the past ready to go: medical tape, two pairs of socks, etc.

Do not try anything new at this point; it is simply not worth the risk.

Do not even think about getting new footwear for race day. Use your trusted old running shoes that you know will not let you down.

When it comes to race day, you will probably be nervous. This is normal, but you should not ever give in to self-doubt! When you cross the finish line, you will have shown "self-doubt" who the boss is!

All of the eating the day before race day will have helped, but you still need to eat a good breakfast. I would advise that you double up on your normal portion size; this should be done first thing and at least an hour before you start.

WHEN YOU SET OFF

As soon as the claxon goes, you will feel a surge of adrenaline—and so will everyone else. This will mean that the overall pace will be slightly faster than most people can handle.

As long as you keep this in mind and stay disciplined, in a few short miles, you will probably be passing the guys that started off too fast.

When you are faced with a twenty-six mile run, the last thing that you want is to be struggling in the early stages.

So when you set off, you should set your pace at least 10% slower than your normal running speed. Let everyone who has been subliminally bitten by the "adrenaline bug" overtake you, and think about your own game at this stage.

A good start will really help to boost your confidence. You can up the pace later if you feel that you can handle it.

Once you are at a comfortable pace, try and make a conscious effort to stick to this. It will be very easy to unconsciously follow other runners and use them as pace makers.

This can work out great, but it can also push you too much. So be aware and remember that this is a marathon, not a sprint. The more comfortable that you can make yourself, the better the whole experience will be.

CHAPTER 24

CONCLUSION

Whether you purchased this book to simply improve your running progress or you actually want to take up the challenge of running a full—or even half—marathon, I believe that the information that has been shared is solid advice, and I have done my best to keep it as simple as possible.

I write from my own fitness experience and back up my theories with the results that I have earned from my own training and I try my best not to overcomplicate things. When I first started running, a one and a half mile run would take me at least fifteen minutes and I would be exhausted. When I reached my peak, I could run the same one point five mile circuit in eight minutes and twenty two seconds. I would also be confident to run a marathon any day of the week.

The information in this book documents some of the most important lessons that I have learned on this journey that enabled me to make this change, so I hope that you find value in the pages and that the information helps you to avoid some of the mistakes that I made, so you get to your finish line that bit quicker.

It is one thing reading and digesting the literature, but it is another thing to take action! It is only this action that will give you the results that you want.

So if you are a total beginner who has never been into fitness or even weight loss, you can utilize this information to get you started. If you feel that this is still too advanced but you would like to eventually run a marathon, no problem!

It is a great start, and your goal is a big one. But it is these big goals and your journey to accomplishing them that will really set you aside as a great achiever.

You may want to check out my beginner fitness book "Home Workout For Beginners". This will give you a very strong foundation to work from.

After the six-week beginner programme outlined in "Home Workout For

Beginners", you will be more than ready to start progressing on to the routines mentioned in here.

If you are already running or training for endurance and long distance, you should be looking to push yourself that little bit more on a regular basis. By taking my advice, you will have the tools for this progression.

I hope that you have enjoyed this book and that it can help you cross many finish lines. And, as always, I am more than happy to give you advice should you need it.

I am always eager to hear what you think of my work. I would really appreciate it if you left a review and rating.

It would be great if you returned to the retail store where you got this from and tell others about your experience. These rankings are driven by readers and customers like you.

If you head over to the store and search for, "Marathon Training & Distance Running Tips," this book page will be displayed.

Please take a few moments to do this if you have enjoyed this book so far.

You can also read the other books that I have mentioned that will compliment this book and help you out further by heading over to my author page on my website

See this series at:

JimsHealthAndMuscle.com

Thanks for the feedback, and I truly wish you all the best with your fitness goals! ☺

Email: Jim@jimshealthandmuscle.com

Good luck and all the best,

Jim

CHAPTER 25

ONE MORE THING

In the following chapter, I am leaving you with an excerpt from another book of mine:

"Fitness & Exercise Motivation"
By
James Atkinson
(Also available on audio and also read by Matt Addis)

This excerpt is very apt for the conclusion of this book, and I hope that it can bring you some motivation and belief in your own ability to smash your fitness goals!

All the best,
Jim

CHAPTER 26

IT STARTS WITH A REASON

Whenever anyone decides to take on a fitness venture, new diet, or healthy lifestyle change, there is always a trigger. If there wasn't a reason to do this, why would it even cross your mind?

Most people who decide that they want to start a physical training routine or health diet will want to do this because of the way they feel. It might be that they feel overweight and unattractive, and when they see themselves in the mirror, they don't like what they see. On the other hand, it might be that they are training for a sporting event and bodily changes need to be made.

The point is; if you are looking to start a new fitness regime, there is always a reason.

Most people, including my past self, overlook this extremely powerful tool called 'Reason' by having a subliminal reason; that is, they don't exactly know what their reason is. This can really weaken their chances of success at the subconscious state.

When I look back on my own personal experiences today, I can identify my reasons for doing the things I did. I can explain my reasoning for the big choices I made. But at some points in my life, I know could not.

I was in my late twenties when I first started to utilize this tool, and it was actually someone else who set me on this way of thinking. I had gone into bodybuilding in a big way since I left the army several years earlier, and I had wanted to compete in a bodybuilding show for the last few years.

One day, I was speaking to a work colleague during break whilst showing him some pictures of some of the guys who trained at my gym and who had already competed in bodybuilding shows. My work colleague didn't have the slightest interest in fitness or physical training, and I should've probably been chatting to him about something else. But when someone has a passion for a goal or a hobby, they tend to share it with everyone they meet, and I had gone very much down this rabbit hole.

As he flicked through the picture gallery on my phone, you could follow his thought process by looking at his face. The subjects of these photographs were of men who were wearing nothing but a set of extra small posing trunks. They were smeared in deep, dark, fake tans with hard, lean, muscular physiques; and to top it off, they were all striking some kind of "show off" pose.

As he handed my phone back to me, with a grimace on his face, he said:

"Why do you want to look like that?"

In my infinite wisdom, I replied in my typical light-hearted style, "Chicks dig muscles, don't they?"

Although my answer didn't do a lot for the reputation of the bodybuilding community, it was, no doubt, the kind of answer that my colleague had come to expect of me, as I am a bit of a joker anyway. It was obvious that he wasn't very impressed with my plans and I realized that the discussion had come to an end, so we steered the conversation in another direction.

On my way home from work that night, when I had plenty of thinking time in my car, I thought about his question again.

Why do you want to look like that?

Now that I was alone with my thoughts, I could be perfectly honest with myself without being scrutinized by anyone but yours truly. So, what were the real reasons?

As I made the forty-five-minute car journey back home, I set about questioning myself and searching to find the real reasons that I wanted to contest in a bodybuilding show. Most people don't want to do this kind of thing so there must be something that had caused me to want to take up the challenge.

After being brutally honest with myself and facing the potentially humiliating truth, I came up with the real reasons. I was able to identify that wanting to compete in a bodybuilding show was a progression from overcoming an inferiority complex that I had when I was in my younger, more influential years, and an unfulfilled need to overcome a physical and mental challenge.

But if I had said that to my work colleague earlier, he would have probably been left speechless as it would have been way out of character for me to confess such a thing. And, in all fairness, earlier that day, I didn't realize that was the answer, either.

When I was younger, I was always a small kid. I really wanted to be the

Johna Lomu or Scott Gibbs on the rugby pitch and destroy my opponents with my awesome power, speed and bulk. When I watched these guys play rugby on television for their respective countries, I developed goose bumps as I watched them knock other players down, break out of multiple tackle attempts and carry the ball across the try line to lead their team to victory. But I would only ever be able to imagine what it felt like to be them. I was too small and weak to be anything but a liability on the rugby pitch, so I had to settle for being a substitute player. Until I found that I could work on my strength and size using a weight-lifting routine!

Many years later, after overcoming many more challenges and learning some valuable lessons along the way that, in turn, shaped my personality and changed me into a different person altogether, I would jump at any opportunity to prove that I could overcome tough physical and mental challenges.

I hit bodybuilding hard, and, after a few years, I actually looked like a bodybuilder. But to really reach my potential, I would have to strip away as much fat as possible, and the only real way to do this is with some solid accountability. What better way to put yourself under pressure to achieve a goal than to have a timescale and strong reason to accomplish that goal. If I were to commit to a bodybuilding competition and the day of the competition finally came, I would be standing on a stage in nothing but a tight thong, and in front of several hundred people. Now, if you were going to be doing that, you would really want to look your best!

On that drive home, I found out a lot about myself and it was as a result of being true to a simple question that my work college had thrown at me.

At that point, I committed to the bodybuilding competition. Although it was only months away, and I could bow out at any time, I decided I wasn't going to. I would see it through to the end and stand on that stage looking the best that I possibly could.

This appears to be the underlying reason that would carry me to the finish line. But there were other powerful reasons working their magic in the background, too:

I was working a job that was not suited to me and really needed a challenge outside of work.

I wanted to push myself to see how far I could go.

I didn't want to be the average Joe who lifted weights and had some size.

I didn't want to be the guy who says, "I thought about doing a bodybuilding show once." I wanted to be the guy who says, "I did a bodybuilding show once, and here's my trophy."

I wanted to add bodybuilding competition to my "Achieved" list.

I had been out of the army for several years and needed the challenge of hardship that comes with competition prep, so that I could taste the sweetest of sweetness after the long months of sour when the competition was over. (This is an awesome feeling!)

I wanted an epic Facebook profile picture ☺

So, as you can see, finding a powerful reason or a number of reasons to take you beyond your own targets to achieve personal victories is not just a surface thought process. To get the best out of this tool, you must delve deep into your soul and really try to hit the nail on the head. And the more honest that you can be with yourself, the more of an accurate truth you will find.

Remember that you are the only person who knows your real reasons for wanting to change your fitness levels; so it pays to be as critical as you can be with yourself. This is how the most powerful reasons come to light.

If the reason isn't strong enough to drive you forward and force you to your feet when the challenges of your goal bring you to your knees, then the reason isn't good enough! Everyone's reasons will be different, and what one person might find ridiculous or even comical, might be strong enough to drive another person past limits beyond their own comprehension.